A Companion to
Aphorisms
&
Quotations
for the Surgeon

Edited by
Moshe Schein

tfm Publishing Ltd, Castle Hill Barns, Harley, Nr Shrewsbury, SY5 6LX, UK.
Tel: +44 (0)1952 510061; Fax: +44 (0)1952 510192
E-mail: nikki@tfmpublishing.com; Web site: www.tfmpublishing.com

Design and type-setting: Nikki Bramhill
First Edition © 2008
ISBN 978 1 903378 61 8

Printed by Gutenberg Press Ltd., Gudja Road, Tarxien, PLA 19, Malta.
Tel: +356 21897037; Fax: +356 21800069.

Contents

Foreword

Since its publication, about five years ago, *Aphorisms & Quotations for the Surgeon* found its place in surgeons' personal and public libraries. It received favorable reviews in surgical journals but what most matters to me is the warm feedback I have received from many surgeons. They told me that the book has been useful to 'decorate' their lectures or manuscripts with relevant 'smart' or 'entertaining' entries. Some like to quote from the book during teaching rounds or conferences. Many simply enjoy it for its collective wisdom and wit. I have observed surgeons browsing the book at one of the surgical meetings, citing to each other one of the quotations and laughing: "how true!"

The original *Aphorisms & Quotations for the Surgeon* included some 1600 aphorisms and quotations. But over the last few years I retrieved and came across a large number of new potential entries; now surgeons tend to send me anything which sounds to them a potential aphorism: "you may want to include it in your next volume" they often write. By 'retrieve' I mean that many of the entries were not written or uttered to serve as stand alone aphorisms, but they were picked up by me from articles and medical and non-medical books. So having collected and selected a fair number of entries which, I think, deserve to be added to the surgeon's intellectual armamentarium, we decided to publish them in a separate, smaller book, to serve as a companion to the first volume.

I have practiced surgery in three continents, in vastly different surgical cultures but noticed that while each has its own 'set' of aphorisms, the surgical truths remain the same. According to Howard Fabing:

Since the days of Hippocrates, our father, the aphorism has been the literary vehicle of the doctor... laymen have stolen the trick from time to time, but the aphorism remains the undisputed contribution of the doctor to literature.

The term 'aphorism' (*aphorismos* in Greek) denotes a 'short, pithy sentence' or a 'concise statement of a principle' or 'a terse and ingenious formulation of a truth or sentiment'. Also, 'rules' and 'quotations' may easily fall under such description. This book, like its preceding 'big brother', brings a medley of over 500 aphorisms, quotations, and rules by surgeons and non-surgeons, about surgery, surgeons and anything which may be relevant to the practice of surgery. I attempted to gratify all potentials tastes - by including ancient as well as contemporary entries, formal and colloquial, pronounced by surgical giants or anonymous - only guided by the prerequisite that the entry appeals to the surgical soul. I attempted, however, to eliminate self-congratulatory and self-righteous clichés - commonly uttered by surgeons who stand up to speak in public.

Karl H. Bauer (1890-1978) wrote: "Show me your favorite aphorism and I will tell you who you are." This would of course apply to this book where I used my editorial prerogative to select some aphorisms and exclude others. This has been pointed out by Dr. Robert E. Condon in his introduction to the previous volume: "Some of Dr. Schein's weltanschauung, despite his prefatory disclaimer, is contained in the collection of aphorisms within the covers of this book." Be it as it may, my purpose was to provide the surgical reader with a source of a large and wide variety of surgical aphorisms and quotations. I am sure that readers will enjoy many of the entries but hate others according to their personal taste. And I hope that readers, especially the younger surgeons, will discover that surgical truth is old, that what they think is a novel idea has been said before, and that what they observe around them has been observed years ago. It may contribute to their humanity and humility, perhaps even add maturity to their surgical personality and practice, and with a bit of luck increase their sense of surgical humor - which in the era of political correctness has tended to dry up.

Moshe Schein
Ladysmith, Wisconsin (2008)
mschein1@mindspring.com
www.docschein.com

Sources

I compiled the entries for this book from multiple sources. Many were sent my way by surgeons from all over the world (after they have seen or read *Aphorisms & Quotations for the Surgeon*); some I gathered from the daily 'online' chat on SURGINET (an international discussion forum for surgeons); a number of entries were cherry picked by me from surgical books, books about surgical history or even novels; current surgical literature or lectures was another source.

If known, the names of those who allegedly coined the entry are provided; when unknown they are not. It is obvious that many aphorisms and quotations simply float around, re-paraphrased in many versions, often claiming originality and under multiple 'authors'. In order to provide historical perspective we added the date of birth and death - if known - of the authors. Authors cited without an accompanying date are hopefully still alive. Clearly, most entries belong to the collective surgical folklore - thus, the property of the eternal surgical community and not deserving a copyright.

Readers who wish to comment or to add entries to the next edition of this book please e-mail me directly: mschein1@mindspring.com.

Acknowledgements

A large number of surgical friends and colleagues around the world provided aphorisms and sources. Many are cited along their contributions. The following deserve special acknowledgement (in random order):

Dr. Leo Gordon: I should add that he is one of the wittiest contemporary aphorists among American surgeons (you have to read his *Cut to the Chase*). Special gratitude to Professor David Dent of Cape Town who is one of my favorite aphorists and Dr. Rick Paul of Amsterdam. I am indebted to Mr. G. Morris-Stiff (UK) for his collection of Ivor Lewis' aphorisms. Many thanks also to Kenneth Mattox, George Bock, Douglas Geehan, Alex Berzoy, Alexander Schoucair, Angus Maciver and other members of SURGINET.

1

Academics

1   Instructors can take a point and explain it. Assistant professors can take a point and turn it into a lecture. Associate professors can take a point and turn it into a course. Professors can take a point and turn it into a career. Deans have forgotten the point.

Lee Reichman

2   A crucial academic rule: do unto others as they would do unto you; only do it first.

2

Acute abdomen

1   [About intestinal obstruction]: It is wholly unnecessary, and dangerous, to wait for an accurate diagnosis. This can be done only by abdominal section, and this had better be done before death than after it.

Robert Lawson Tait, 1845-1899

2   Acute intestinal obstruction is diagnosticated by exclusion (e.g. of peritonitis). Its seat [large or small bowel] is fixed by injection [i.e. enema]. Its variety is determined by its seat and the age, antecedents and symptoms of the patient. Its treatment is surgical on or after the third day, if the symptoms are urgent and forced injections fail.

Benjamin Heber Fitz, 1843-1913

3   All these operations [for intestinal obstruction] are of the gravest type and yet too often, chiefly because of the seniority system in our hospitals, they are undertaken by young and inexperienced men.

C. J. Miller, ~1929

4   With abdominal distension, expect vomit at any time.

Ivor Lewis, 1895-1982

5   Some patients instead of being too sick to be operated are too sick not to be operated.

3

Amputations

1

L'amputation chirurgicale d'un membre est l'oevre la plus philosophique de toutes les sciences humaines: Surgical amputation of a limb is the most philosophical work of all human sciences.

Pierre Dufouart, 1737-1813

4

Anatomy

1   The student should endeavor to prevent the bad effects of sitting for hours in a cold dissecting room; the most effectual way is to put on an additional flannel jacket, and carpet shoes over his boots... a cap should be worn in preference to a hat, which is not only inconvenient, but also quickly acquires a bad smell.

John Hunter, 1728-1793

2   The right lung consists of three parts... Klotchkov raised his eyes to the ceiling, striving to visualize what he had just read. Unable to form a clear picture of it, he began feeling his upper ribs through his waistcoat.

Anton Chekhov, 1860-1904

3   The diaphragm is a muscular partition that separates disorders of the chest from disorders of the bowels.

Ambrose Bierce, 1842-1914

4   Every anatomic part has a function, and if you think of its purpose it's easier to remember where it is and what it looks like.

George Crile, Jr, 1907-1992

5   Anatomy is something everyone has, but it looks better on a girl.

Bruce Raeburn

6   Beware the four birds of the chest: i) vagoose, ii) esophagoose, iii) azygoose, iv) thoracic duck.

5

Anesthesia

1   My hands are then henceforth, washed of chloroform and devoted to ether.

James Marion Sims, 1813-1883

2   There is an amazing transformation that occurs when an anesthetist leaves the state sector for private practice. It is transformation from obstruction to grovel. In the private sector they clean the surgeon's shoes, and anaesthetize anyone or anything.

David Dent

3   It is usually a bad sign if the anesthesiologist is asking you if you are losing a lot of blood during a case especially when you're not.

Michael Hoffman

4   It is usually a bad sign if there are three or more anesthesiologists in the operating room at the same time and none of them is reading the newspaper.

Michael Hoffman

5   The definition of an anesthetist by surgeons: a half-asleep doctor who is taking care of a half-awake patient. The definition of a surgeon by anesthetists: someone trying to disturb the sleep of the patient.

Ahmad Assalia

6   An epidural is a needle you put in a woman's back that makes her numb from the waist down… for years.

Chip Franklin

6

Appendicitis

1   The appendix serves and protects the cecum from rupture by too great an accumulation of 'superfluous wind' because it has the ability to dilate and contract.

Leonardo Da Vinci, 1452-1519

2   Theoretically it would seem to be much better if we would cut down upon the appendix as soon as the diagnosis was tolerably certain..., tie it above the seat of perforation, and remove from its neighborhood any concretion or decomposing material that might be the cause of irritation.

Samuel Fenwick, 1821-1902

3   Humans can survive easily without an appendix, but surgeons can do so only with difficulty.

Rudolph Virchow, 1821-1902

4   If, after the first twenty-four hours from the onset of the severe pain, the peritonitis is evidently spreading, and the condition of the patient is grave, the question should be entertained of an immediate operation for exposing the appendix and determining its condition with reference to its removal. If any good results are to arise from such treatment it must be applied early.

Benjamin Heber Fitz, 1843-1913

5   [In acute appendicitis]: If delay seems warranted, the resulting abscess, as a rule intra-abdominal, should be incised as soon as it becomes evident. This is usually on the third day after the appearance of the first characteristic symptoms of the disease.

Benjamin Heber Fitz, 1843-1913

6   I hope I may never again go everyday to visit a threatening case [of acute appendicitis] waiting bashfully for the authority of a clearly defined peritonitis before I dare take action.

Charles McBurney, 1845-1913

7   Purgation means perforation; in an appendix kinked and bad; food and drink worry him; and aperients drive him mad.

John Blair Deaver, 1855-1931

8   We also know that a diseased appendix may express itself through some other mouth-piece and become confused with organic disease of the stomach or the duodenum or the intestines. By reflex action it may cause spastic contractions of the pylorus, pylorospasm, giving rise to symptoms purely gastric in character; or it may affect the secretion and cause the so called secretory neuroses...

John Blair Deaver, 1855-1931

9   I have sometimes been misled to open the abdomen in the presence of predominantly gastric symptoms, only to find the pyloric sphincter to be the seat of spasm of toxic or reflex appendiceal irritation, as evidenced by the complete relief of symptoms following appendectomy.

John Blair Deaver, 1855-1931

10   The only causes of chronic appendicitis are: i) actinomycosis, ii) tuberculosis and iii) remunerative.

Ivor Lewis, 1895-1982

11   [About interval appendectomy]: To prevent its recurrence [of acute appendicitis]... we had removed Jane's appendix, a prophylactic procedure that was popular in those days. Today I would never recommend it. Now we have antibiotics.

George Crile, Jr, 1907-1992

12   Mesenteric adenitis is code for: I thought it was appendicitis, but the appendix was normal.

David Dent

13   The proportion of perforated appendicitis is not a good measure of quality. The proportion of perforations may increase because you operate on fewer patients with non-perforated appendicitis. A high proportion of perforations may in fact be a good thing because it means you operate only on those patients who need surgical treatment.

Roland Andersson

14   If a patient has right lower quadrant pain and no appendectomy scar, put one there.

Rip Pfeiffer

15   It is not true that the appendix is worthless - it has put thousands of surgeons in expensive cars.

7

Art

1   The art of medicine consists of amusing the patient while nature cures the disease.

François-Marie Arouet de Voltaire, 1694-1778

2   Surgery is both an art and science. The science is pretty straightforward. The art influences the discipline in many ways, some of which border on the mystical.

Leo A. Gordon

3   When physicians talk about the 'art of medicine' they usually mean healing, coping with uncertainty, or calculating their deferral income taxes.

Frederick L. Brancati

4   What you can do for a patient is infinitely more important that what you can do to a patient. The art of surgery is to discover the difference.

Robert Flemma

8

Assessment

1   A little look saves a lot of talking.

Ivor Lewis, 1895-1982

2   Never study an improving situation.

Leo A. Gordon

3   Never allow a patient (unattended) near an interventional radiologist on a Friday afternoon, at night or during a weekend.

Leo A. Gordon

4   Last year's study, reportedly 'normal' is always abnormal.

Leo A. Gordon

5   The emergency room is the best place to evaluate an emergency.

Leo A. Gordon

6   The quality of the X-ray ordered is directly proportional to the specificity of the clinical information supplied to the radiologist.

Leo A. Gordon

7   The test for fitness for operation is the ability of the patient to walk to the operating room.

Andy Gage, Sr

8 The road to the operating room does not always have to pass through the CT scanner but an indicated CT may obviate the need for an operation.

M. S.

9

Assistants & Residents

1 If I ever deliberately commit murder I shall select an inattentive and awkward assistant as my victim. I shall select one who has assisted enough to delude himself into thinking he could himself do the work better than the surgeon who is operating. This usually reaches the high point at about the third week of the intern's experiences.

Arthur E. Hertzler, 1870-1946

2 The chief activity of an incompetent assistant is to try and do the operation.

Arthur E. Hertzler, 1870-1946

3 There are no better assistants than nurses. Their only thought is to assist the surgeon. This implies, of course, that there were no young doctors about.

Arthur E. Hertzler, 1870-1946

4 I must repeat again that operative surgery is learnt by assisting. Close attention to a technical master, while assisting him, makes the master's technique a second nature, and the real teacher of operative surgery, by having his assistant occasionally complete one stage of an operation, sometimes another, will give the pupil adequate confidence in his own power and a feeling of competence greater than that of the man who is too early left on his own.

Ian Aird, 1905-1962

5 [To a resident]: I'd hate to think that when I was at your stage, I was this slow.

Angus B. McLachlin, 1908-1987

6   When residents answer a question with a question they almost certainly do not know the answer.

Mark M. Ravitch, 1910-1989

7   Resident involvement in an operation is earned. It must be clarified and delineated before the procedure begins.

Leo A. Gordon

8   The attending surgeon is always right. Residents who follow this rule are assured of excellent resident evaluations, glowing letters of recommendations and perhaps a future partnership position.

Leo A. Gordon

9   [To residents during the operation]: My grandmother can operate better than you... and she's DEAD. [Or], I prayed to God for help with this operation... and He sent me YOU! [Or], We started out with a beautiful operation, and you've turned it into THIS! [Or], These are dark days in surgery.

Bill Wall

10   An assistant who cannot see the problem can rarely help with the solution.

Rick Paul

11   A poor assistant is better than a talented opponent.

Rick Paul

12   Scut... forgive me for this; I HATE this word. Ward work is patient care. It's the work of angels and saints. It is a privilege to do. It's fun. It is necessary to the care of patients. If you call this patient care scut, you (and your protégés) won't do it. If you call an admission a hit, you won't take care of them. Your language defines your feelings. Your feelings determine what you have energy for. I get energy from getting a patient a cup of coffee, drawing their blood well, and closing their skin in a nice manner... as much energy as I get from transplanting their hearts and lungs, and bypassing their vessels. I can't do what I don't have energy for.

Curt Tribble

13   [To the assistant]: It's OK to move... surgery is a mobile sport.

Bruce Schirmer

10

Biliary & Liver

1 [About the first portocaval shunt in dogs]: I consider the main reason to doubt that such an operation can be carried out on human beings has been removed because it has been established that the blood of the portal vein, without any danger, could be diverted into the general circulation.

Nikolai Eck, 1849-1917

2 Thus with stone obstruction of the duct: dilation of the gallbladder is rarely observed; the organ has already undergone contraction; with obstruction from other causes, dilation is to be expected; atrophy exists only in 1/12 cases.

Ludwig Courvoisier, 1843-1918

3 An intra-operative cholangiogram is a religion - not science.

Nathaniel J. Soper

4 Beware of the easy looking gallbladder and the overconfident surgeon.

11

Bleeding & Hemostasis

1   If it were not for the frightful hemorrhage which so frequently attends them, operations would be robbed of nearly all their terror, and few men would shrink from their performance.

Samuel Gross, 1805-1884

2   Rules for sudden haemorrhage: i) be calm, ii) clamp or pack, and iii) adequate exposure and deal as necessary.

Ivor Lewis, 1895-1982

3   You can tell how bad the surgeon is by the stink of the Bovie in his OR.

Douglas Geehan

4   I love the smell of the Bovie in the morning - it is the smell of victory.

Allan Siperstein

5   Bleeding in the belly is like fire on a ship - you run towards it.

Jeffery Young

6   Bleeding started in the rectal area and continued all the way to Los Angeles.

A patient's chart

7   DIC = deep in chit.

12

Breast

1   We are now dissecting the axilla and having a terrific time with the intricacies of the brachial plexus. I would never have dreamed after watching breast cancer operations that there were so many things there.

George Crile, Jr, 1907-1992

2   ... there is no basis for advocating any single type of operation for operable cancers of the breast, and there is no basis for employing a general policy, pro or con, regarding irradiation, removal of the endocrine glands or endocrine therapy. Surgery, irradiation and endocrine therapy are double edge swords that harm as well as help. The challenge to the surgeon is to control the cancer as well as possible and to do so with least possible harm.

George Crile, Jr, 1907-1992

3   There was never a Tuesday or a Friday on which Yevgenia Ustinova did not cut off women's breasts and she would remark to the orderly who cleaned the theatre, a cigarette between her exhausted lips, that if all the breasts she cut off were collected together and made into a pile the result would be quite a little mountain.

Alexander Solzhenitsyn

4   Asya brought it (her breast) close to his face and held it for him. 'Kiss it! Kiss it!' she demanded... he nuzzled it with his lips like a suckling pig, gratefully, admiringly... its beauty flooded him... Today it was a marvel. Tomorrow it would be in the trash bin.

Alexander Solzhenitsyn

5   Beware a lumpy area that does not feel right and images as normal.

Michael Dixon

6   A typical breast cancer is easy to diagnose - it is the atypical one in a young patient that causes diagnostic problems.

Michael Dixon

7   The battle is between margins and cosmesis and we must think like the 'oncoplastic' surgeon.

Marvin J Silverstein

8   Breast doctors are usually called Monica or Kimberley, having a web site with help page, a clinic with flowers, plants and statuary, a public grouping raising money, and the shrill insinuation at large meetings that XYs were mutilating women and this must stop!

David Dent

9   The medical profession can invent tests for breast disease faster than they are found out to be useless.

David Dent

10   Failure to diagnose breast cancer is one of the most common reasons for physicians to be sued in the US. One must remain suspicious, but still use some common sense. Sometimes you can't do both.

John Kennedy

11   Never assume that there is payback for time spent. Lengthy discussion of intraductal carcinoma, lobular carcinoma *in situ* and other controversial areas result in the proper surgical procedure scheduled and performed expertly... by someone else!

Leo A. Gordon

13

Cancer surgery

1   Leaving the least part of the cancer is equal to leaving the whole.

John Hunter, 1728-1793

2   We shall never overcome cancer by surgery: it will be something we shall inject.

George Grey Turner, 1877-1951

3   [About the American Cancer association]: Those responsible telling the public about cancer have chosen to use the weapon of fear. They have bred in a sensitive public a fear approaching hysteria. They have created a new disease, cancer phobia, a contagious disease that spreads from mouth to ear.

George Crile, Jr, 1907-1992

4   Alas, lymph nodes do not DETERMINE prognosis, they are merely MARKERS of prognosis. No one with gastric carcinoma ever died from lymph nodes. The lymph nodes are the footprints in the snow of where the cancer has already been, and has passed on. Sweeping away footprints is futile.

David Dent

5   We are only at the foothills of understanding cancer, and the biological mountain still lies in the clouds ahead.

David Dent

6   There are more people living off cancer than are dying from it.

14

Colorectal

1   The doctor should put his finger into the anus of this patient and if he finds within something as hard as a stone... this is certainly a tumor. Often it erodes and consumes the whole circumference of [the anus, and] it may never be cured with human treatment.

John of Arderne, 1306-1390

2   [Anal] fissures are small and painful ulcers, following the whole length of the bottom wrinkles, resembling chilblains of the lips or hands; they are caused sometimes by the hardening of faeces...

L. G. Lemonier, ~1689

3   The examining physician often hesitates to make the necessary examination because it involves soiling his finger.

William J. Mayo, 1861-1939

4   Rectal examination must not be neglected in diagnosis... I do not mean instrumental but digital examination. This procedure is so repulsive to both physician and patient that it is readily passed by... [to omit it] is criminal where the suspicion of obstruction has arisen.

Ernest Amory Codman, 1869-1940

5   Sounds that might shock a duchess are music of the spheres to the surgeon.

William Heneage Ogilvie, 1887-1971

6   Small town surgeons often prefer to send them to the local tertiary centers for the 'subtotal colectomy for colonic inertia' as opposed to 'backwoods slash-artist chopping out constipated colons'. Been there.

Angus Maciver

7   A rigid proctoscope made in 1935, when properly used to detort a sigmoid volvulus, can do more than any GI fellow with a $50,000 model x-6700 three-chip video laser-CD-ROM triply-enhanced surround-sound colonoscope.

Leo A. Gordon

15

Colostomy

1   [About colostomy]: But I much question the propriety of such an operation... since if the patient survives he must become... loathsome to himself and to those around him.

B. W. Brown, ~1853

2   Failure of a colostomy closure is more due to the youth of the colostomy than the youth of the surgeon.

Ivor Lewis, 1895-1982

3   If you think about a colostomy, you should do a colostomy.

Leo A. Gordon

4   There is no law that says that a colostomy must be closed.

Leo A. Gordon

16

Complications

1

Nothing stands out so conspicuously, or remains so firmly fixed in our memory, as something in which we have blundered.

Cicero, 105-43 BC

2

The complication most to be feared is pneumonia; this can often be avoided, if I may put it this way, by giving atropine... and placing the patient on an open porch where he can have the benefit of plenty of fresh air. I have not found the administration of oxygen in these circumstances of much service; indeed, it is apt to be harmful, as it often is annoying to the patient and interferes with sleep.

John Blair Deaver, 1855-1931

3

With sudden postoperative collapse, the cause is much more likely to be a surgical complication than 'medical.'

Ivor Lewis, 1895-1982

4

Of course I love you darling; I'll send you the money by the next mail; I never see fistulas.

Dick van Geldere

5

Those patients seen on rounds do not need to be seen on rounds. Those patients missed on rounds have manifestations of an early surgical complication that could be detected on rounds.

Leo A. Gordon

6   [As to *schadenfreude*]: The thrill of avoiding a complication that has befallen a colleague insures that your patient will experience the same complication within two weeks.

Leo A. Gordon

7   The rule of '2': when you hear a surgeon telling his number of performed cases, divide it by two. When he tells about his complication rate, multiply it by two.

Rick Paul

8   Beware a surgeon who is an expert in managing complications.

9   Avoid iatrogenesis fulminans.

10   No matter what you do, the number of complications will be double if a patient or his spouse is either a physician or a nurse.

11   An ounce of prevention is worth a pound of cure.

17

Conservatism

1   Let man learn to be honest and do the right thing or do nothing.

James Marion Sims, 1813-1883

2   A good surgeon is a doctor who can operate and knows when not to operate.

Theodor Kocher, 1841-1917

3   The doctor employing expectant treatment has only the satisfaction of knowing that he is doing nothing injurious - a merit... that is today sometimes overlooked.

Arthur E. Hertzler, 1870-1946

18

Consultation

1   The usual procedure for a doctor when he reached the patient's house was to greet the grandmother and aunts effusively and pat all the kids on the head before approaching the bedside.

Arthur E. Hertzler, 1870-1946

2   Any case presented as: "See the patient when you can at your convenience" is a four-plus-flat-out surgical emergency with a mortality rate of 98% and should be seen immediately.

Leo A. Gordon

3   Use humor with patients and families judiciously - you must stop all attempts at humor after the first blank look.

Leo A. Gordon

19

Controversy

1   Everything is controversial in surgery, always was, always will be.

2   Even if something stops to be controversial there will always be some stupid muzik who will claim it is controversial.

3   What was controversial before, and is not controversial anymore, will become controversial again very soon.

4   Any list of surgical controversies from the 1950s can form a basis of a current discussion: we know more and controversies remain.

5   Increasing knowledge fuels new controversies.

6   The more medical options we have, the more advanced is the technology, the more are the controversies.

20

Death

1 Stop lying! You know, and I know, that I am dying. So do at least stop lying about it!

Leo Tolstoy, 1828-1910

2 We never save anyone's life, for life, itself, is a fatal disease.

Paul C. Bucy, 1904-1992

3 Rather let the patient die in peace, than in pieces.

Dr. Frascani

4 Death: irremediable breakdown between a patient and doctor.

Martin Winckler

5 Even an in-growing toenail operation has a hundred percent mortality - eventually.

6 Every neurotic patient ultimately dies of organic disease.

21

Diagnosis

1   You cannot operate on a differential diagnosis.

Claude Organ, Jr. 1926-2005

2   When all else fails, order a physical exam.

Leo A. Gordon

3   A living problem is better than dead certainty.

4   The most important thing to remember about rare diseases is that they are rare.

22

Drains

1   The more imperfect the technique of the surgeon the greater the necessity for drainage.

William Stewart Halsted, 1852-1922

2   Never ask the following questions: Would you drain it? Should you drain it? Did you drain it?

Leo A. Gordon

3   That you call something a drain does not guarantee that it actually drains.

Rick Paul

23

Drugs

1   One should drink vodka, though. It acts as a stimulant on the brain, which, flabby and inert with continual movement, makes one stupid and weak.

Anton Chekhov, 1860-1904

2   The patient will always be given a drug to which he is allergic (but) the administration of that drug will have no effect.

Leo A. Gordon

3   Acute, *adj*: something that occurs without warning. As is the pain one gets when approached by a drug rep at the end of a busy day.

Howard Bennett

4   Medical rep: person who gallantly camps in the waiting room in order to throw some light on the doctor's consultation and leaves him freebies to be used for treating his mother, wife and children.

Martin Winckler

5   Pharmacist: medical auxiliary whose main field of competence, acquired through long experience, is to know how to decipher and translate prescriptions, and whose main function is to sell shampoos, toothpastes and slimming creams. In tubes.

Martin Winckler

6   The patient on steroids will walk for you to the morgue.

24

Education

1   Never let formal education get in the way of your learning.

Mark Twain, 1835-1910

2   It may well be counted among the joys of the surgeon to train worthy successors in the work he loves so well.

John Blair Deaver, 1855-1931

3   I have never yet been able to understand why undergraduates are exposed to clinics in major surgery... before these operations become important to them a long apprenticeship is, or should be, required. I learned in (medical) school all the little details in the technique of abdominal hysterectomy, but no one thought to tell me not to molest the little boils which sometimes form in the upper lip.

Arthur E. Hertzler, 1870-1946

4   When I review my own professional life and its many satisfactions, the greatest are not the surgical operations I have performed, nor the thousands of patients that I have cured, but the successful young surgeons whose instruction and training I have directed.

George Heuer, 1882-1950

5   The young surgeon who, during his pursuit of a research problem, has learned to operate with safety upon a dog, is a surgeon to whom operations in man can be trusted.

Owen H. Wangensteen, 1898-1981

6   The young surgeon who learns the basic precepts of asepsis, hemostasis, adequate exposure and gentleness to tissue has mastered his most difficult lessons.

Robert M. Zollinger, 1903-1992

7   Could you fix my glasses, please, let's see how your surgical skills are.

Kenneth W. Warren, 1911-2001

8   One way to understand surgical residency training is as a set of rites, rituals and ordeals designed to transform outsiders into insiders, laypersons into professionals.

Charles Bosk

9   It is essential among such groups that elitism, although almost an anachronism in modern times, be raised as an emblem rather than dropped apologetically.

Seymour Schwartz

10   A poor surgeon hurts one person at a time. A poor teacher hurts 130.

Mary J. Wilson

11   The public exposure of surgical ignorance is the true path to the public exposure of surgical brilliance.

Leo A. Gordon

12   You teach yourself surgery and I will teach you how to think as a surgeon.

Leo A. Gordon

13   Today medical school is attended by mobs, not students; mob receives its degree, a doctor-mob practices the medical profession. We learn to distrust it immediately; this mob may ever be armed, may even be equipped with powerful weapons.

Guido Ceronetti

25

Empathy

1   The ability of the old doctor was enhanced because he remained at the patient's bedside until his suffering was relieved, even though it required many hours to achieve that end. While so engaged the doctor learned much about the nature of the illness.

Arthur E. Hertzler, 1870-1946

2   The individual on whom we operate is more than a physiological mechanism. He thinks, he fears, his body trembles if he lacks the comfort of a sympathetic face. For him nothing will replace the salutary contact with his surgeon, the exchange of looks, the feeling that the doctor has taken charge, with the certainty, at least apparent, of winning.

René Leriche, 1879-1955

3   No physician, sleepless and worried about a patient, can return to the hospital in the midnight hours without feeling the importance of his faith. The dim corridor is silent; the doors are closed. At the end of the corridor in the glow of the desk lamp, the nurse watches over those who sleep or lie lonely and wait behind closed doors. No physician entering the hospital in these quiet hours can help feeling that the medical institution of which he is part is in essence religious, that it is built on trust. No physician can fail to be proud that he is part of his patient's faith.

George Crile, Jr. 1907-1992

4   A good trick is to remind yourself from time to time that the family you are talking to could be yours.

James Rucinski

26

Errors

1   [There is] a tendency always to attribute fatalities... to sins of omissions, whereas the many evi
results of the sins of commission are given much less consideration.

J. L. Yates, ~1905

2   One can survive anything nowdays except death.

Oscar Wilde, 1854-190(

3   All bad outcomes can be traced backwards in time to a series of mistakes and stupid things
we did that in summation led to 'deep shit'. Except being hit by a meteor... that is fate. All else
starts with something stupid.

Paul Zaveruha

4   Most 'avoidable' surgical mortalities are not caused by one - sentinel - horrendous, clearly
evident - error which cries "I am malpractice." Instead, most such 'avoidable' deaths result
from a chain of allegedly 'minor' hesitations, confusions, ignorance, greed, inattention,
overconfidence, arrogance, stupidity - which together drive the nails into the coffin. Taken
together they may whisper: "we are negligence..."

M. S.

5   To err is human. To forgive is against departmental policy.

27

Ethics

1   Anyone who proposes to do good must not expect people to roll stones out of his way, but must accept his lot calmly if they even roll a few more upon it.

Albert Schweitzer, 1875-1965

2   In order to have a constant stream of referrals, the surgeon must please the referring physicians. Sometimes this is best accomplished by doing what those physicians approve or want done. When these desires run contrary to the best judgment of the surgeon, conflicts of interest again appear. If the surgeon does what he thinks his colleagues expect, he may not be doing what he believes is in the best interests of his patients.

George Crile, Jr, 1907-1992

3   My primary professional goal has always been: to get sick people well, and when that has proven impossible, to add to their comfort until the end.

Kenneth W. Warren, 1911-2001

4   I pledge to be always myself and never pretend to be what I am not or do what I cannot; I pledge never to play God, and never to be generous with other people's money; I pledge never to indulge in the delusion that, as a physician, I have stronger will and lesser needs than 'normal' people, for I will be able to understand and help the sick and the weak only if I accept my own sickness and weakness; and if I breach this pledge, may I not become a great and famous doctor.

Antonio E. M. Attanasio

5   I think that a man is doing his reporting well only when people start to hate him.

V. S. Naipaul

28

Experience

1 Experience can also consist of doing the same wrong thing over and over again.

Dick van Geldere

2 Experience is what you rely on when you haven't read anything for a while.

Howard Bennett

29

Feeding

1   [On American nutrition]: Even what they eat and drink, these palefaces who don't know what wine is, these vitamin-eaters who drink cold tea and chew cotton-wool and don't know what bread is, these Coca-Cola people... their pink sausage skin, horrible, they only live because there is penicillin... their fake health, their fake youthfulness.

Max Frisch, 1911-1991

2   If I need grape sugar, give it to me through the mouth! Why this twentieth century gimmick? Why should every medicine be given by injection? You do not see anything similar in nature or among animals, do you? In a hundred years' time they'll laugh at us and call us savages...

Alexander Solzhenitsyn

3   There is no way a patient is going to eat a hole in the anastomosis.

P. O. Nyström

4   Do you mean that you start your patients on a clear liquid diet and then progress to a full liquid diet before a regular diet? If so, this is a silly practice that should be ceased. It is all solid shit when it goes through the anastomosis so who cares how it starts.

Karen Draper

30

Feelings

1   Complacency and smug satisfaction are danger signals of decadence, just as wholesome discontent and healthy introspection and self-criticism are indications of the will and desire for improvement.

John Blair Deaver, 1855-1931

2   A physician is obligated to consider more than a diseased organ, more even than the whole man - he must view the man in his world.

Harvey Williams Cushing, 1869-1939

31

General concepts

1   Surgery is the best of the medical sciences; less liable than any other to the fallacy of conjectural or inferential practice; perpetual in its applicability; the worthy produce of heaven and the certain source of fame.

Dhanwantaree, ~600 BC

2   A work on surgery... without principles, may be compared to a vessel at sea without helm or rudder to guide it to its place of destination.

Samuel Gross, 1805-1884

3   In the craft of surgery the masterword is simplicity.

Berkeley Moynihan, 1865-1936

4   The fourth dimension in surgical management is time.

Ivor Lewis, 1895-1982

5   Surgery is not difficult, nor scary, it is fun.

Kenneth W. Warren, 1911-2001

6   Practice of gentleness to tissue is more important than the preaching... but the technique of an operation should be regarded as only a small part of the total care of a patient.

Kenneth W. Warren, 1911-2001

7   The right man in the right spot of the right time means life or death to the fortunate or poor patient.

Marian Littke

8   Surgery is a performing art. It better be good. The patient takes the repercussions of the act, the nurses watch the actual show and the pathologist writes the criticism.

P. O. Nyström

9   Surgery is the last of the true blood sports.

Wilson Carswell

10   Never answer an unattended ringing medical center telephone.

Leo A. Gordon

11   Every effect has a cause; Euclid stated this long ago. Spontaneous and idiopathic are medical code words for 'don't know'.

David Dent

12   Never refer to an operation as 'just a…'. It reflects lack of appreciation for surgical pathology. For any procedure in surgery can result in horrible complications. The vagaries of human biology assure this.

Leo A. Gordon

13   When in doubt, you take it out, and if you can't wait, you operate.

Ernie Palanca

14   Outcome of surgery depends on: 96% preparation, 1% execution (i.e. the doing of it), 1% repetition, 1% clean-up (for our nursing sisters), 1% luck.

Tom Gilas

15   General advice in treating patients: don't scratch where it doesn't itch.

Rick Paul

16   Winning is overemphasized. The only time it is really important is in surgery and war.

Al McGuire

17   High risk diseases should have low risk operations.

32

Giants & Greatness

1   Never ask me what I have said, or what I have written, but if you will ask me what my present opinions are, I will tell you.

John Hunter, 1728-1793

2   [When accused of altering his views from one year to the next]: very likely I did. I hope I grow wiser every year.

John Hunter, 1728-1793

3   I know, I am but a pigmy in knowledge. Yet I feel as a giant, when compared with these men.

John Hunter, 1728-1793

4   It has always been the fate of those who have illustrated the arts and sciences by their discoveries to be beset by envy, malice, hatred, destruction and calumny.

Leo Augengrugger, 1772-1809

5   A great surgeon cannot be recognized by the public. They have no way of judging between a good doctor and a quack or between a real surgeon and a mere pretender.

Augustus Charles Bernays, 1854-1907

6   Halsted is an obsessed fuddy-duddy who takes all day to do an operation that should never be done at all.

George Washington Crile, 1864-1943

7   The master surgeon declares his class, not only by his operating expertness but by his understanding of the entire situation.

Arthur E. Hertzler, 1870-1946

8   A Cowboy's Guide to Life: Always drink upstream from the herd.

Texas Bix Bender

33

Glory & Fame

1   In looking back upon his early career it is difficult for a surgeon to say whether his trials overshadow his triumphs or vice versa.

John Blair Deaver, 1855-1931

2   The profession of medicine and surgery must always rank as the most noble that men can adopt. The spectacle of a doctor in action among soldiers, in equal danger and with equal courage, saving life where all others are taking it, is one which must always seem glorious, whether to God or man.

Winston S. Churchill, 1874-1965

3   What is now known as Lembert's suture, which ensures that serous surface is applied to serous surface in suturing intestine, is the foundation of all modern gastric and intestinal surgery, and the inventor (Antoine Lembert, 1802-1851) of this suture deserves more prominence than is usually given to him.

Zachary Cope, 1881-1974

4   As a surgeon I am no longer afraid of my failures, for success is nothing but failure turned inside out.

Samir Johna

5   If you do not come up on a google.com search you are a nobody.

M. S.

34

Hands & Manual skills

Funktionslust is the desire to perform a technical procedure because we perform it well... it refers to the joy and pride from performing a skill well. The accomplished musician, the skilled athlete, the ballerina, and the skilled surgeon are all justifiably proud of their skills and usually have a love for practicing their art. But *Funktionslust* can also be a curse. It can be a temptation to do a larger procedure, where a smaller simpler procedure would suffice. *Funktionslust* may prevent a surgeon from learning a new technique that appears to be less satisfying in terms of the pure joy of operating. *Funktionslust* may be a factor in a surgeon's failure to refer a patient to another specialist: for non-surgical treatment or for a different surgical procedure.

Roger S. Forster

35

Heart

1   It is infinitely better to transplant a heart than to bury it to be devoured by worms.

Christian Barnard, 1922-2001

2   [About the first human heart transplant]: It was a natural progression of open heart surgery. We did not think it was a great event and there was no special feeling. I was happy when I saw the heart beating again. We did not stand up or cheer or something like that. I didn't even inform the hospital authorities that I was going to do the operation.

Christian Barnard, 1922-2001

3   The Wright brother's first flight was shorter than a Boeing 747's wing span. We've just begun with heart transplants.

C. Walton Lillehei

4   A car mechanic said argumentatively to his client, a cardiac surgeon: "So Doc, look at this work. I also take valves out, grind 'em, put in new parts, and when I finish this baby will purr like a kitten. So how come you get the big bucks, when you and me are doing basically the same work?" The surgeon replied: "Try doing your work with the engine running."

Legend has it that the Doctor was Michael DeBakey

5   Pericardiocentesis: aptly termed a needle with a clot at each end.

36

Hemorrhoids

1   Hemorrhoids are swellings of the orifice of the anal veins, forming granulations, and frequently letting blood flow out.

Celsus, 25BC-AD50

2   [Treatment of hemorrhoids]: Force out the anus as much as possible with the fingers and make the irons red hot, burn the pile until it be dried up and so that no part may be left behind.

Hippocrates, 460?-377? BC

37

Hernia

1   If one considers the operations which they [the ancient surgeons] performed it will be found that they would operate on all those hernias which were not strangulated, whilst we only operate on those in which strangulation puts the patient in peril of his life.

Jean Louis Petit, 1674-1750

2   I am not the only one who has observed that operations for herniae which are not strangulated have not such happy results as those which are done for strangulated herniae.

Jean Louis Petit, 1674-1750

3   What is the use of opening the sac? I know of none except to explore the intestine and omentum, to remedy complications if there are any.

Jean Louis Petit, 1674-1750

4   No altered or mortified part should be returned loose to the belly.

Percival Pott, 1714-1788

5   It is a most unpardonable neglect on the practitioner not to use tobacco [enema] in strangulated hernia, which ought to be impressed on every surgeon.

Astley Cooper, 1768-1841

6   To record even cruder general results of so many operations (~1000) for the repair of inguinal hernia are required special training, some zeal and a particular honesty of purpose.

William Stewart Halsted, 1852-1922

7   I have no failure to record, if we exclude the recurrences which I have reported and which could not be ascribed to my method.

William Stewart Halsted, 1852-1922

8   The surgeon is fortunate and likely to be true to himself whose observations are controlled by mature assistants with large experience in the operative treatment of hernia and who are as eager as he to ascertain and state the exact truth.

William Stewart Halsted, 1852-1922

9   A surgeon can do more for the community by operating on hernia cases and seeing that his recurrence rate is low than he can by operating on cases of malignant disease.

Sir Cecil Wakely 1892-1979

10   Hernia repairs are like sex... you have to do what works best for you, with the minimum of complaints afterwards.

Angus Maciver

38

History

1   The only thing we ever learn from medical history is that we never learn.

John B. McKinlay

2   When I was younger, I always told the residents that the first sign of senility in a surgeon is when he demonstrates an interest in surgical history.

Leo A. Gordon

39

Incisions

1   When the doctor is in doubt and the patient in danger, make an exploratory incision and deal with what you find as best as you can.

Robert Lawson Tait, 1845-1899

2   The decision is more important than the incision.

3   Midline is the incision of indecision.

40

Infection

1   Suppuration may be considered a resolution but it is a mode of resolution which we mainly wish to avoid.

John Hunter, 1728-1793

2   If I had the honour of being a surgeon, I would never introduce into a human body an instrument that had not been passed through boiling water and better yet a flame, just before an operation, and rapidly cooled.

Louis Pasteur, 1822-1895

3   When it had been shown by the researchers of Pasteur that the specific property of the atmosphere depends on minute organisms, it occurred to me that decomposition in an injured part might be avoided by applying as a dressing some material capable of destroying the life of the floating particles.

Joseph Lister, 1827-1912

4   Humanity has but three great enemies: fever, famine, and war. Of these, by far the greatest, by far the most terrible, is fever.

Sir William Osler, 1849-1919

5   Even diseases have lost their prestige, there aren't so many of them left. Think it over... no more syphilis, no more clap, no more typhoid... antibiotics have taken half the tragedy out of medicine.

Louis-Ferdinand Celine, 1894-1961

6   A surgeon should never be satisfied with himself nor with the others as far as asepsis is concerned.

Robert Danis, 1880-1962

7   Prophylactic antibiotics will turn a third class surgeon into a second class but will never turn a second class surgeon into the first class one.

Owen H. Wangensteen, 1898-1981

8   The greatest boom to surgery's advance in this century has been control of cellulitic infections through chemotherapeutic agencies, the sulfonamides and antibiotics. When will surgery experience another great catalytic forward thrust like that achieved through anesthesia, prophylactic antisepsis, and the antibiotics?

Owen H. Wangensteen, 1898-1981

9   [On necrotizing fasciitis]: [His] leg was monstrously swollen, the skin was stretched tightly without a single wrinkle, and it filled all his ample trouser leg. Right up to his hip the skin had gone a shiny dark-violet hue and was covered with spots velvety to the touch. Similar spots, only of a lighter tinge, had made their appearance on his swarthy, deeply sunken belly. A foul, putrescent stench came from the brown blood dried on his trousers...

Mikhail Sholokhov, 1905-1984

10   The advent of antibiotics has greatly lowered the incidence of hand and other infections, opened the way for prophylactic treatment, and reduced the need for surgical drainage. However, over the years one theme has recurred: initial care is pre-eminent in the prevention and treatment of all surgical infections.

J. J. Byrne

11   Historically, the most common errors in usage include the widespread use of antibiotic prophylaxis in clean surgery and the faulty timing of administration. The most common error today [in the use of prophylactic antibiotics in surgical practice] is continuation of the agents beyond the time necessary for maximal benefit.

Ronald L. Nichols

12   Nietzsche once stated, "That which does not kill you only makes you stronger." While he was not necessarily referring to bacteria and their relationship to antibiotics, the quotation nonetheless applies.

Mikaela Chilstrom

13   The headline reads, "Docs say patients make them prescribe useless antibiotics." This puts a physician in roughly the same predicament as a serial killer. The latter says, "Stop me before I kill again, while the former says, "Stop me before I prescribe again."

Nicolas Martin

14   Pus is like the truth - you have to let it out.

Gareth Morris-Stiff

15   Sepsis is a slight upon surgical virility.

John Alexander-Williams

16 La mierda y la sangre no ligan. (Shit does not mix with blood.)

Rolando Ramos

17 In peritonitis, operating on a poorly resuscitated patient is like throwing both ends of the rope at a drowning man.

41

Innovations & Gimmicks

1

In these days when science is clearly in the saddle and when our knowledge of disease is consequently advancing at a breathless pace, we are apt to forget that not all can ride and that he also serves who waits and who applies what the horseman discovers.

Harvey Williams Cushing, 1869-1939

2

... Many pints of fluid were used to wash out the abdominal cavity. Some surgeons appeared to attribute their successful results to the thoroughness of their washing-out. It did not take many years, however, to find out that this prolonged washing-out was quite unnecessary in the case of perforated ulcer, and very harmful in the case of a perforated appendix. Yet it was some time before the custom was entirely dropped. It was a common custom when first I begun my medical studies... [but] when it was found that irrigation with antiseptics was harmful, and with otherwise harmless fluids like saline solution quite unnecessary, then washing-out was abandoned.

Zachary Cope, 1881-1974

3

If the life of a scientific fact is seven years, the life of a favorite treatment is half of that.

George Crile, Jr, 1907-1992

4

The paradigm shift in surgical truths was from vehemence-based and eminence-based medicine, to evidence-based medicine.

David Dent

5

First it was the abolition of acid reductive operations for peptic ulcers, then it was not operating on diverticular disease, then not operating on knobby goiters, but investigating them, and now it's this stenting outrage. Our surgical parents had to put up with the abolition of the superior mesenteric artery syndrome, and colectomy for constipation in low spirited ladies, and sympathectomy for just about every form of vascular disease, and phrenic nerve crush for asthma. There is a sustained assault on the livelihood of surgeons, but happily they can invent operations faster than they are found out to be useless. Laparoscopy is re-finding old operations and is working on new ones by some form of laparoscopic hitching, stapling or removing - for bloating, queasiness, gluttony, or general lowness of spirit.

David Dent

6   How do you diagnose bile leak after NOTES cholecystectomy? By a bitter taste in the vagina.

Herman Smith

7   Be not the first by whom the new is tried, nor yet the last to lay the old aside.

8   When technology is the Master, the result is Disaster.

42

International surgery

1   There are really three great training systems in surgery, the British, the American and the Continental European. Each of these has its advantages and, each two of the three would admit of the third, its disadvantages. It is remarkable that, differing as they do, all three systems manage to produce the same kind of elite and the same kind of honest-to-God workaday surgeons.

Ian Aird, 1905-1962

2   I was through with accepting as gospel what American surgeons taught, and I was ready to explore other branches of science that might be of use in my practice. I also wanted to see in other countries what other surgeons had discovered. I no longer felt that American surgeons, whether at Harvard Medical School or the Cleveland Clinic, had the answers to all questions.

George Crile, Jr, 1907-1992

3   The words of Tolstoy's Cossack, Yeroshka, who said about West European doctors: "All they can do is cut. Well, they're fools. But in the mountains you get real doctors. They know about the herbs."

Alexander Solzhenitsyn

4   Surgery is what a surgeon practices. An operation is what a surgeon performs. In this context, there is no such word as surgeries. In Great Britain, surgeries are treatment rooms. Neither an operation nor a patient is a case, but that's another commentary.

C. J. Allen

5   I hope this helps your sister-in-law unless the Yank surgeons have already yanked her to the OR!

Deepak Chatterjee

6

Reimbursement: complex system for racketeering, laundering and recycling money between a producer (pharmaceutical laboratory), wholesaler (pharmacist), dealer (physician) and drug consumer (the insured person) under the supervision of two nationwide criminal organizations (the French State and pharmaceutical industry).

Martin Winckler

43

Intestine

1   In ileus the belly becomes hard, there are no motions, the whole abdomen is painful, there are fever and thirst and sometimes the patient is so tormented that he vomits bile... Medicines are not retained and enemas do not penetrate. It is an acute and dangerous disease.

Hippocrates, 460?-377?, BC

2   [About intestinal obstruction]: ...cometh with constipation of the belly and busy costing [vomiting] and the huge acheing and sorrow, as though the guts were bored with wymball [gimlet]... and the matter that should pass out beneathenforth cometh out the mouth.

John of Arderne, 1306-1390

3   Would it be not better to make an incision and draw out the strangulated intestine with fingers, than leave the patient in danger of his life?

Paul Barbette, 1632-1704

4   This [anastomotic] method is equally applicable to all solutions of continuity of the intestine and even the stomach; its technique will be the same though it may assume a different form.

Antoine Lembert, 1802-1851

5   [About intestinal anastomosis]: The uniform continuity of the peritoneal surfaces, and the ready disposition of these surfaces to assume the adhesive inflammation, are the means provided by nature for the reparation of intestinal wounds and injuries.

Benjamin T. Travers, 1783-1858

6   In cases of intestinal obstruction, when the physician's art has failed to give relief, the surgeon's aid is occasionally requested and it would be well for the medical mind to recognize that in a large proportion of cases this aid is sought too late a period.

Thomas Bryant, 1824-1914

7   Intestinal adhesions are the refuge of the diagnostically destitute!

Sir William Osler, 1849-1919

8   Occlusion of the mesenteric vessels is regarded as one of those conditions of which the diagnosis is impossible, the prognosis hopeless, and the treatment almost useless.

A. Cokkins, ~1921

9   Subjects with acute intestinal obstruction die from the phenomena of septic poisoning.

Frederick Treves, 1853-1923

10   The suggestion that radiography should be employed in the diagnosis of intestinal obstruction is one which should be condemned whole-heartedly... I prefer the seeing eye of a living human clinician to the scientific eye of a dead machine.

H. J. Paterson, 1932

11   It is now accepted by everybody that the chief cause of death in simple obstruction of the small bowel... is circulatory failure due to loss of water and electrolytes.

W. D. Gatch & C. G. Culbertson, ~1939

12 Scout films taken 8 or 24 hours after a half ounce of oral barium are invaluable in managing intestinal obstruction.

Ivor Lewis, 1895-1982

13 It is obvious from the physiological consequences that if all patients with mechanical obstruction are operated upon as soon as the diagnosis is made, the operative mortality will be high. If there are signs of ischemia, immediate operation is indicated, otherwise allow time to replenish water and electrolyte deficits.

G. Thomas Shires, 1925-2007

14 The truth is that most patients [with early postoperative intestinal obstruction] will improve without you ever knowing whether it was a mechanical obstruction or 'just' an ileus.

M. S.

44

Judgment

1   For every problem there is one solution which is simple, neat and wrong.

Henry Louis Mencken, 1880-1956

2   It is the surgeon himself who must take the final decision, and in making it he necessarily stands apart from his colleagues in a kind of loneliness.

Ian Aird, 1905-1962

3   The hardest thing about being a surgeon is knowing when not to do something. Some people don't understand that, but it is the most important thing. The natural tendency is, or course, to do something, to take action. It really comes down to judgment, which most people don't think of as a surgical skill.

Norman M. Kenyon

4   Intuition is the fastest way to reach a wrong solution.

Dick van Geldere

5   When common sense interferes with a protocol, follow common sense.

Leo A. Gordon

6   In the overwhelming majority of instances a therapeutic decision was arrived at in direct relation to what happened in the last similar case the doctor was familiar with.

Lucien L. Israel

7   Know what you will do in the event you don't know what to do.

Rick Paul

8   The supreme surgeon uses his supreme judgment to avoid situations that would test his supreme abilities.

9   Judgment is not the act of making a snap decision. Judgment is like playing chess... You need to think three or four moves ahead.

10   Here lies Sir Archibald Arbuthnot Slagg-Heepe FRCS - seldom correct, but never in doubt.

11   It takes only a few years to learn when to enter the abdomen but many years to learn when to stay out.

45

Laparoscopy

1   Human mind like parachute; works best when open.

A Chinese proverb

2   Laparoscopy has a definitive role in cases where the trauma of incision is greater than that of excision.

48

Military surgery

1   To perform a task as difficult as that which is imposed on a military surgeon... I am convinced that one must sacrifice oneself, perhaps entirely, to others; must scorn fortune and maintain an absolute integrity and must inure oneself to flattery.

Dominique Jean Larrey, 1766-1842

2   It is necessary to begin always with the most dangerously injured, without regard to rank or distinction.

Dominique Jean Larrey, 1766-1842

3   It is important for the head surgeon to study well the countries that the armies cross, in order that he might know to benefit the injured using resources that localities can offer.

Dominique Jean Larrey, 1766-1842

4   No matter how cruel an operation may be, it is an act of humanity in the hands of the surgeon when it may save the life of the injured; and the greater and more immediate the danger, the more the aid must be prompt and energetic... in this circumstance the man of the art does his duty and never thinks about his reputation.

Dominique Jean Larrey, 1766-1842

49

Money matters

1   Beware of patients who call you 'Doc.' They rarely pay their bills.

William Osler, 1849-1919

2   If the doctor is good - people will feed him, if the doctor is bad - we don't need him.

N. Semashko, Soviet Minister of Health, ~1930

3   Economic considerations sometimes motivate the physicians to accept that part of the scientific evidence that best supports the method that gives him the most money.

George Crile, Jr. 1907-1992

4   Training, practice, and economic pressures can push the surgeons' thinking in the direction of more frequent, more radical, and more remunerative surgery. It is not that surgeons consciously decide to do an operation for economic reasons. The decision is more subtle, and is based on training and on habits of practice which through the years have been influenced by economic pressures, always in the same direction. If there is a question between operating or not operating, it is economically sound to operate. If it is a question of a big operation or a little one, it is better economically to do the big one. If it is a question of surgery versus radiation, it is surgery that gives the advantage to the surgeon. Finally, if it is a question of doing the operation oneself or referring the patient to a better-qualified specialist, it is obvious that there is little profit to be derived from referral.

George Crile, Jr. 1907-1992

5   I am sure that one of the reasons why salaried physicians and surgeons are apt to be the first to adopt simplified methods of treatment is that unlike those in private practice, their income is not directly affected when the treatment is less costly.

George Crile, Jr, 1907-1992

6   Don't let cost-containment become care-containment.

Leo A. Gordon

50

Morbid obesity & Bariatric surgery

1   Severe obesity restricts the movements and maneuvers of the body. It compresses blood vessels causing their narrowness. Breathing passages are obstructed and the flow of air is hindered leading to nasty temperament... on the whole these people are at risk of sudden death... they are vulnerable to stroke, hemiplegia, palpitation, diarrhea, fainting... any physical effort they make will weaken them.

Avicenna, 980-1037

2   [Minimal invasiveness] for patients is now such a matter of fashion that patients would prefer to have a less effective, micro-invasive procedure rather than a mini-invasive, more effective procedure, which is in my opinion simply idiotic.

Nicola Scopinaro

3   Bariatric surgeons should inhabit a special place in Hell, where they are condemned to repair the hernias they have created.

Angus Maciver

51

Nursing

1   Constant attention by a good nurse may be just as important as a major operation by a surgeon.

Dag Hammarskjold, 1905-1961

2   Doctor, ever' year I get hundreds of applications fouh internship heuh, but I have a helluva time keepin' nurses. Yuh will try to get along with 'em, wont ya?

Alfred Blalock, 1899-1964

52

Old patients

1 The test for fitness for surgery in geriatric patients is to pull a sheet over their faces, and if they pull it down - they are fit!

David Dent

53

Old & young surgeons

1   Surgeons of old experience... consciously or subconsciously long for the day when they shall do their last operation.

Arthur E. Hertzler, 1870-1946

2   The old surgeon... knows that the mortality published as two percent, at best, is such only in the hands of the most experienced operators, and finally most likely the statistics are wrong.

Arthur E. Hertzler, 1870-1946

3   A young surgeon should keep his affections in cold storage.

Ian Aird, 1905-1962

4   "The young physician starts life with 20 drugs for each disease, and the old physician ends life with one drug for 20 diseases," said **William Osler (1849-1919)**. Similarly, the greenhorn surgeon knows about numerous surgical options for each condition but when aging he adheres to the one option that he can do best.

M. S.

5   For surgeons an old man is somebody ten years older than you.

Avi Roy Shapira

6   And middle-of-the-night aneurysms never failed to leave his nerves jangling like a steel band on speed. As a young man he could cat-nap on a washing line, yet be instantly awake and alert when necessary, but now at fifty-eight, his old bones took longer to settle and even longer to spring into action.

Mike Albany

7   It just wasn't exciting anymore. At sometime over all those years, surgery had become a production-line treadmill: hernias, gallbladders, colons, veins, stomachs, breasts... when did it happen?

Mike Albany

8   Then there were the on-calls, like tonight. Thirty years ago it was every other night and his body could cope with it easily; now it was only once a week and every fifth weekend, but the constant stone-in-the-shoe feeling of waiting for the phone to ring always left him drained.

Mike Albany

9   What to do with the competent but physically limited old surgeons? Make them administrators - they'll still make mistakes, but won't cause any bleeding.

Andy Gage

10   Incompetence does not necessarily come with age - generally, the incompetent physician was that way from the start of his career. What comes with age is stiff fingers, perhaps a tremor, less visual acuity and diminished endurance, losing technical skills as a result.

Andy Gage

11   Be kind to people on the way up so they will be kind to you when you are on the way down.

54

Operating room

1   But if another gives (...instruments), he must be ready a little beforehand, and do as you direct.

Hippocrates, 460?-377?, BC

2   It is remarkable that during the four or five years, when as an operator, I wore them [gloves] occasionally, we could have been so blind as not to have perceived the necessity for wearing them invariably at the operating table.

William Stewart Halsted, 1852-1922

3   The operating room is the surgeon's laboratory.

William Stewart Halsted, 1852-1922

4   The patient undergoing an operation is peculiarly vulnerable to infection. It is desirable, therefore, that the theater suite should be physically separated from the rest of the hospital.

Sir John Loewenthal, 1914-1979

5   Is there any way you can be of help in this operation, besides leaving the room?

Michael E. DeBakey

6   Leave your attitude outside the operating theatre.

Leo A. Gordon

7   The first rule for the operating room visitor is: get permission from the operating surgeon before speaking.

Leo A. Gordon

8   Never refuse 7.30 operating time.

Leo A. Gordon

9   The number of supplies and instruments a surgeon says he'll need is inversely related to the amount he will ultimately require.

Patty Swenson

10   In the operating room we can save more lives, cure more cancers, restore more function, and relieve more suffering than anywhere else in the hospital.

R. Scott Jones

11   Many lives have been saved by a moment of reflection at the scrub sink.

Neal R. Reisman

55

Operating (technical)

1   All instruments ought to be well suited for the purpose in hand as regards their size, weight, and delicacy.

Hippocrates, 460?-370?, BC

2   [About using the anastomotic button he invented]: It takes about as long to describe the operation as to perform it.

John B. Murphy, 1857-1916

3   The actual manipulative part of surgery requires no very great skill and many an artisan shows infinitely more adeptness in his daily work.

Frederick Treves, 1853-1923

4   The rituals of an operation commence before, sometimes long before, the incision is made, and may continue for a long period after the wound is healed.

Berkeley Moynihan, 1865-1936

5   Studying pathology or post mortems gives a rough hand... orthopedic surgery give a rougher one... keep your feather-edge touch-stick to straight surgery.

George Washington Crile, 1864-1943

6   The poky operators sometimes excuse themselves on the grounds of thoroughness.

Arthur E. Hertzler, 1870-1946

7   If an operation is difficult, you are not doing it properly.

Robert E. Gross, 1905-1988

8   Staplers are not a quick road to surgery for the untrained and will not turn a neophyte into a virtuoso.

Mark M. Ravitch, 1910-1989

9   **Michael Hobsley** used to say, before starting a parotidectomy, "take the clock down, nurse, and put a calendar up."

10   It's not practice that makes perfect. It's perfect practice that makes perfect.

Vince Lombardi

11   Go to the heart of danger and there you will find safety.

Kenneth L. Mattox

12   Tie a suture like you embrace the one you love: firmly but tenderly.

Rick Paul

13   Big mistakes are made through small holes.

Rick Paul

14   In my humble opinion dissection with the hook is like eating soup with a fork.

Pieter Prinsloo

15　[Murphy's laws for surgeons]: If anything can go wrong, it will. If it looks easy, it will be difficult. If it looks difficult, it will be damn near impossible. If everything seems to be going well, you probably overlooked something.

Steven W. Merrell & James M. McGreevy

16　It is my understanding that the stapler is rarely to be blamed in mishaps. The surgeon has the greater share of blame. The learning curve about staplers is about not asking the stapler to manage situations beyond its capacity and applicability.

P. O. Nyström

17　A Cowboy's Guide to Life: If it don't seem like it's worth the effort, it probably ain't.

Texas Bix Bender

18　Six Ps: proper planning and preparation prevents poor performance.

19　If you do not know what you are cutting, don't cut it!

20　When you don't know what you are doing: be extremely careful.

56

Other specialties

1   Only by standing at the elbow of the surgeon, let me repeat, can the internist hope to attain proficiency in diagnosis and proper... treatment...

John Blair Deaver, 1855-1931

2   Accustomed to legerdemain and quick results [the surgeon] is apt to regard the diagnosis and treatment of a headache, for example, as a trivial matter, forgetting that the internist may require hours of probing before discovering that what the patient needs is not a new pair of glasses but a new mother-in-law.

Thomas Findley, ~1944

3   Loeb's laws of medicine: If what you're doing is working, keep doing it; if what you're doing is not working, stop doing it; if you don't know what to do, don't do anything; above all, never let a surgeon get your patient.

Leo Loeb, 1869-1959

4   We surgeons tend to dive into the swamp and look around for alligators while our internist colleagues analyze the swamp water for its osmolarity, acidity, and nutrient contents to see if the water will support life. We are plungers, they are lanners.

Alden H. Harken

5   You recognize a surgeon or an ob-gyn because he has blood on his shoes, a urologist because he has urine on his, and an anesthetist because on his you see spots of spilled coffee.

Bernard Cristalli

6   If the gynecologist says it is not adnexal it is always adnexal.

Leo A. Gordon

7   What is the advantage of a man over a woman? He will never need to be operated on by a gynecologist!

Victor Bruscagin

8   Ortho surgeons usually think that the heart's job is to pump antibiotics to their joint replacement.

Mark Hamilton

9   Surgeons believe that anything with fiber optics on one end should have a surgeon on the other.

Edward Thompson

10   Going to a male gynecologist is like going to an auto mechanic who never owned a car.

Carrie Snow

11   When medicine docs try to talk you into doing high risk surgery always be wary of the courage of the non-combatant.

Matt Wahl

12   Surgery is the red flower that blooms among the leaves that are the rest of medicine.

Richard Selzer

13   Why are gastroenterologists more imaginative and courageous than us surgeons in employing new and bizarre invasive therapeutic modalities? Because they have somebody (us) to bail them out!

Eli Mavor

57

Pain

1   Doctors when they get sick... howl louder than the common run and are just as much interested in their own private pain, the interest in which completely overshadows their scientific training.

Arthur E. Hertzler, 1870-1946

2   When the primary indication for an operation is pain, that's what you'll get.

Mark M. Ravitch, 1910-1989

3   If you are afraid to hurt the patient, you are going to KILL the patient.

Tom Curry

4   Surgeons don't have to get on their hands and knees and beg the nurses to stop writing useless crap in the chart long enough to please, please, please bring some pain medicine.

Karen Draper

58

Pancreas

1 It is fascinating to conjecture how an inflammatory process in a retroperitoneal gland can produce abnormalities in so many organs.

Reginald Fritz, ~1889

2 The surgeon cannot intelligently operate on organs of double function without a full knowledge of their internal and their external secretions, for here may lie the cause of the failure of a mechanically well executed operation to cure the patient.

William J. Mayo, 1861-1939

3 The most common errors in the surgical treatment of acute pancreatitis are to operate too early in the course of the disease, and to do too much, or in the secondary or septic phase of the disease, to operate too late and to do too little.

Kenneth W. Warren, 1911-2001

4 White wine causes pancreatitis. Red wine, cirrhosis.

Maurice Mercadier, 1917-2002

5 I tell patients that the pancreas is like somebody's wife: she doesn't need a reason to be pissed off and, once she is, you had better just lay low and not touch her until she feels like being in a better mood.

Karen Draper

6 Whether you will develop severe pancreatitis or not depends on the quality of what you drink and the amount of *zakuski* you consume.

A Russian surgeon

7   Even if you like and admire your pathologist as I do mine, you cannot give him your full trust when it comes to pancreatic biopsies.

Michael Trede

8   Ductal adenocarcinoma of the pancreas is an incurable disease.

Michael Trede

9   Surgeons operating on pancreatic cancer today can be classified into three groups: the 'aggressive-radical' surgeon who will always attempt major extirpative procedures with resection of major vessels and vascular reconstruction; the 'nihilist-timid' surgeon who avoids getting involved in complex time-consuming risky procedures; and the 'rational' surgeon who will tailor the operation to the stage of the disease, and the patient's general condition and ability to tolerate the operation.

Jackie T. Tracey & Abdool R. Moosa

59

Pathology & Physiology

1   Patients die not of pathological anatomy but the physiological consequences of it.

William Osler, 1849-1919

2   I can make a surgeon out of a physiologist provided he can make surgeons more physiological.

Dallas B. Phemister, 1882-1951

3   Pathologists are always right, just one day too late!

Miles J. Jones

4   Do not create pathology in an attempt to define pathology.

Leo A. Gordon

60

Patients

1   [When undergoing surgery]: Console yourself with the reflection that you are giving the doctor pleasure and that he is getting paid for it.

Mark Twain, 1835-1910

2   It is more important to know the patient who has the disease, than to know the disease that has the patient.

William Osler, 1849-1919

3   With seriously ill patients, one third of the treatment is for the relatives.

Ivor Lewis, 1895-1982

4   The intimacy between patient and surgeon is short-lived, but closer than between a son and his own father.

Alexander Solzhenitsyn

5   For the patients the last doctor is always the smartest doctor.

Leo A. Gordon

6   There are no difficult operations, only fat people.

Stephen Clifforth

7   Never refer to a patient as an organ or as an operation.

Leo A. Gordon

8   The stronger the family ties (helpful and unhelpful) the more intense will be the family's reaction (helpful and unhelpful).

Neal R. Reisman

61

Politics

1   My fellow creatures of the Hospital are a damn'd disagreeable set. The two heads are as unfit for the employment, as the devil was to reigne in heaven.

John Hunter, 1728-1793

2   I will not say it is a disgrace to be a surgeon to St. George's Hospital; but I will say that the surgeons have disgraced the Hospital.

John Hunter, 1728-1793

3   Surgeons in one town knew little or nothing of surgeons elsewhere. A surgeon from Manchester had never visited an operation theatre in Leeds, nor had ever been asked in consultation. As a consequence it was not infrequent to have to listen to disparagement of one surgeon by another; and jealousies, openly expressed, were too often heard.

Berkeley Moynihan, 1865-1936

4   Never turn down a hospital committee appointment and once appointed, never go.

Owen H. Wangensteen, 1898-1981

5   Only a sailor, not a clerk, should be running the ship.

Ivor Lewis, 1895-1982

6   Don't let the bastards get you down.

Jerrald Shaftan

7   Current chiefs of surgery are CEOs not Chief Educational Officers.

Leo A. Gordon

8   I had no place to go; I only knew where not to remain.

Thomas Starzl

9   The *New England Journal of Medicine* reports that 9 out of 10 doctors agree that 1 out of 10 doctors is an idiot.

Jay Leno

10   Trying to get care by a properly credentialed surgeon will be like going to a Chinese restaurant: sorry, no Peking Duck today, and no surgeon on call with thoracic privileges.

Harold Kent

11   Medicine is like the food chain: internists are herbivores - like cattle they bunch and coexist with each other; surgeons are carnivores - if put together they would eat each other.

Joseph P. Holt, III

12   Popular people do not make good leaders. Decisive people with judgment, who are not afraid to tell other people who don't have such good judgment that their judgment isn't very good, make good leaders.

Bobby Knight

13 A Cowboy's Guide to Life: If you get to thinkin' you're a person of some influence, try orderin' somebody else's dog around.

Texas Bix Bender

14 A Cowboy's Guide to Life: Never miss a good chance to shut up.

Texas Bix Bender

15 A Cowboy's Guide to Life: The biggest troublemaker you'll probably ever have to deal with watches you shave his face in the mirror every morning.

Texas Bix Bender

16 In the old days, if you were black and with some IQ and ambition, you were 'Chairman material' - today it is true if you are a woman.

17 At the M & M - like in Brooklyn courts - lie or die!

62

Postoperative care

1   Every surgeon should himself supervise the postoperative treatment.

John Blair Deaver, 1855-1931

2   After the operation the first and most important considerations are: to control pain; to provide for the proper amount of sleep and to guard against complications.

John Blair Deaver, 1855-1931

3   When will these items [gastric aspirate and urinary output] be recorded on the face sheet of all hospital records for the orientation of the surgeon?

Owen H. Wangensteen, 1898-1981

4   When is a surgeon (not a new, but an experienced one) nervous? Not during operations. But basically a surgeon's nervousness being after the operations, when for some reason the patient's temperature refuses to drop or a stomach remains bloated and one has to open it not with a knife, but in one's mind, to see what had happened, to understand and put it right. When time is slipping away, you have to grab it by the tail.

Alexander Solzhenitsyn

5   We now call Intensive Care 'Normal Care' and the Wards 'No Care'.

Stephen Clifforth

6   The operation is over when the patient is eating a cheeseburger and can't remember your name.

Leo A. Gordon

7 The law of discharge: any labs done on the day of discharge will be abnormal.

63

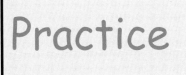

1   Don't drive a nicer car than your referral base does.

Tom Mahany

2   A surgical office referral never generates a surgical case.

Leo A. Gordon

3   You can expect as many referrals to be church-based as medically-based. Whether the problem lies in your specialty or not.

Tom Mahany

4   Fun is a concept rapidly disappearing from clinical medicine today. All of our many detractors do their best to eliminate fun from our profession.

Leo A. Gordon

5   The likelihood that a surgical case will remain in your office is inversely proportional to the amount of office energy expended in arranging that case.

Leo A. Gordon

6   Agreeing to do additional cases when already stretched to meet personal obligations should not be judged as laudable over-achieving. Over-scheduling should instead be understood as a lapse of judgment.

James W. Jones

7   Don't confuse a good result with good practice.

Tom Curry

64

Research

1   When doctors, statisticians and scientists become ill, they ask "Who is the best doctor for this problem?" and not "Which multi-centre controlled trial would be best for me?"

E. J. Freireich

2   A major danger to human health is a young surgical researcher murdering dogs in the basement to develop new operations.

David Dent

3   Any study that reports a certain number of consecutive cases without a complication (death) actually means that the number of cases plus two were performed with two complications (deaths); the first and last.

Michael Hoffman

65

Rural

1   The country doctor's memory was record of the grieves of the countryside as a whole.
Arthur E. Hertzler, 1870-1946

2   The small town needs the best and not the worst doctor procurable. For the country doctor has only himself to rely on: he cannot in every pinch hail specialist, expert, and nurse. On his own skill, knowledge, resourcefulness, the welfare of his patient altogether depends. The rural district is therefore entitled to the best-trained physician that can be induced to go there.
Abraham Flexner, 1866-1959

3   The cost of new devices and training for new procedures is too overwhelming for rural or community hospitals where they have neither the patient load nor the money to invest in new equipment.
Richard M. Stava

4   For some rural physicians a good surgeon is one from whom your patient always returns with one of his abdominal organs missing. A bad surgeon is one who does the opposite.

5   Another rural law: as long as the patient has an appendix, a gallbladder, a uterus and two ovaries, you refer him to the local surgeon. Once these organs are gone you refer to the university.

6   The common perception is that mortalities after an operation in a rural hospital are because "of the inexperienced surgeon or poor care" while if the patient dies in the Ivory Tower then he dies despite "the best efforts of the excellent doctors in the great hospital."

7   [About managing acutely injured patients in US rural hospitals]: If you ship them away they'll accuse you of laziness, cowardice, or losing income for the hospital, but if you treat them locally they'll accuse you of being a 'cowboy' or endangering the patient.

66

SICU

1 Surgical patients no longer die of their primary disease, rather they die of their response to that disease... [thus]... interventions against infection will not alter the course of the disease process whose pathophysiology reflects the response to infection.

John Marshall

2 Principles of intensive care: air goes in and out; blood goes 'round' and 'round'; oxygen is good.

Robert Matz

67

Specialist

1   No man can be a pure specialist without being in the strict sense an idiot.

George Bernard Shaw, 1856-1950

2   A specialist must always appear to be fond of the general practitioner in the same way a good citizen is fond of his dog or the Mountie is fond of his horse.

Ian Rose, ~1960

3   High volume physicians may perform a procedure better, but the patient may have been less likely to need it in the first place.

Robert H. Brook

4   Getting a second opinion is like switching slot machines.

Jimmy Townsend

5   ... it is difficult for a specialist to see beyond his own field, and easy for him to believe that his own particular services are required.

Joseph A. Jerger

6   The primary goal of all generalists is to save patients from specialists.

68

Speed

1 There is no time to think. There is only time to do or let die.

William D. Haggard, 1872-1940

2 A few couples of years spent in the dissection room will save time in the later years by increasing operating speed.

Arthur E. Hertzler, 1870-1946

3 Prolonged operation... is due to lack of anatomical knowledge, making the operator fearful to do long arm strokes and sharp dissection so indispensable to clean and rapid operating.

Arthur E. Hertzler, 1870-1946

4 One time Dr. John Homans [1836-1903], Associate Professor at Harvard and author of *Homans' Surgery*, is said to have passed through Cheever's [David Cheever, 1831-1915] operating room at 8:30 as Cheever was starting a mastectomy. At noon, as Homans passed by again on his way to lunch, he told Cheever, "Hurry up, David, or it will metastasize."

George Crile, Jr, 1907-1992

5 Every case takes as long as it takes and is the only case in the whole world while it is going on.

Bob Crochelt

6   Like fishermen or lovers surgeons are rarely honest about their performance - including operative time. To any surgeon estimation on how long it takes him to perform a procedure: double the time, add 10 minutes for each glass of red the night before, subtract 5 minutes for each year of experience of the assistant, and add 12 minutes for each attractive scrub nurse, and female anesthetist (male if you are a female surgeon), divide by the personal coefficient of efficiency, and finally add 5 minutes for each hour over 6 of operating time that day.

Barry Alexander

69

Standard of care

1 We know that many practicing physicians are not using well proven interventions or implementing well-publicized national guidelines. The legal definition of standard of care protects these physicians and encourages them to change slowly, if at all.

Daniel Merenstein

2 The good thing about a standard of care is that there are so many to choose from.

70

Statistics

1   When anyone essays to publish statistics it impresses me in the same way as when someone
starts to relate a fishing experience. One must admit that the truth is theoretically possible.

Arthur E. Hertzler, 1870-1946

2   Meta-analysis is to analysis as metaphysics to physics.

H. Harlan Stone

71

Stomach, Duodenum & Esophagus

1   [On esophageal perforations]: When it [occurs] it can be recognized but it cannot be remedied by the medical profession.

Herman Boerhaave, 1668-1738

2   The gastric juice is a fluid somewhat transparent, and a little saltish or brackish to the taste.

John Hunter, 1728-1793

3   As to the type of operation [for perforated peptic ulcer], much depends on the state of the patient and upon the experience of the surgeon. The occasional operator may have to contend himself with simple suture of the perforation, but the more experienced surgeon, will, if he is wise, add a gastro-enterostomy and thus ensure better results; while the specialist in abdominal surgery may even venture resection or pyloroplasty...

John Blair Deaver, 1855-1931

4   [In perforated peptic ulcers]: It must be remembered that the exudate in the early cases is sterile or nearly so, and the peritoneal reaction is a response to chemical irritation by the gastric and duodenal contents rather than the result of bacterial invasion.

John Blair Deaver, 1855-1931

5   I believe that peptic ulcer is undoubtedly developed by a combination of local chemical effects, possibly causing prolonged vessel spasm or claudication, a counterpart of Raynaud's disease or scleroderma, or by direct interference with the circulation through infarction by emboli of bacteria, chemically and mechanically active in the tissues and thereby lowering the local resistance to the action of digestive fluids.

Charles H. Mayo, 1861-1939

6   It may really be a compliment to acquire a peptic ulcer; the great genius, the poet, the philosopher are always the most susceptible.

George Washington Crile, 1864-1943

7   Any foreign body which traverses the cricopharyngeus will negotiate the rest of the gastrointestinal tract.

Ivor Lewis, 1895-1982

8   Longstanding pyloric obstruction invariably leads to lengthening of the duodenum, making closure easy.

Ivor Lewis, 1895-1982

9   No [gastric] suction is required after a Polya gastrectomy whilst after a Billroth gastrectomy continue only until bile appears on nasogastric suction.

Ivor Lewis, 1895-1982

10   The esophagus is a difficult surgical field... for its inaccessibility, its lack of serous coat, and its enclosure in structures where infection is especially dangerous and rapid.

Ivor Lewis, 1895-1982

11   Esophagus: as a result of the muscle being loosely knit, anastomosis implies suturing the unsuturable...

Ivor Lewis, 1895-1982

12   Patients with GI disease have GI symptoms.

Larry C. Carey

13   The history of gastric surgery is littered with interpositions, pouches, and attempts to make the gastric reconstruction similar to the underground railway in Vienna.

David Dent

14   Those who *always* do a Billroth II never learned how to do a Billroth I.

M. S.

15   With proper Kocherization you can bring the duodenum through the mouth - and by dividing the lesser omentum and the gastrocolic omentum you can bring the stomach out the ass. Thus, if you want you can do a Billroth I between your stomach and my duodenum without tension - so why do a Billroth II?

M. S.

16   After proximal gastrectomy with esophagogastric anastomosis the reflux is such that the patients lean over to kiss their wives, with green bile running down the corners of their mouth, like blood does from Dracula's.

David Dent

72

Surgeons

1

He is a good surgeon who possesses courage and presence of mind, a hand free from perspiration, tremorless grip of sharp and good instruments, and who carries his operation to success and to the advantage of his patient, who has entrusted his life to the surgeon. The surgeon should respect the absolute surrender and treat his patient as his own son.

Susrata, 800 BC?

2

A barber surgeon... is a man who is sufficiently dexterous to wield the razor when he cuts a beard or open an abscess. A person who is skilful with his hands, no more. A performer. As soon as the act extends to the inner organs... instructions and control can come only from the physicians.

William Harvey, 1578-1657

3

He showed interest in trifles, joked... and chatted carelessly, as a famous surgeon confident that he knows his job will often chat while he tucks up his sleeves and puts on his apron, and the patient is being strapped to the operating table. "I have the whole business at my fingertips, and it's all clear and definite in my head. When the time comes to set to work I shall do it as no one else could, but now I can jest, and the more I jest and the cooler I am the more hopeful and reassured you ought to feel, and the more you may wonder at my genius."

Leo Tolstoy, 1828-1910

4

If the surgeon has risen to the place of social and professional equality with the so-called internists, it is because he has ceased to be a mere mechanician.

John Blair Deaver, 1855-1931

5   The surgeon like the poet is born such.

John Blair Deaver, 1855-1931

6   The surgeon... is a man of action. He lives in an exhilarating world of knives, blood, and groans. His tempo is of necessity rapid. He is inclined to look at his less kinetic colleague with an air of puzzled condescension but may, in a relaxed moment, admit that the medical man is occasionally able to assist uncomfortable dowagers in the selection of a cathartic.

Thomas Findley, ~1944

7   It was generally accepted opinion... that drunken doctors were very capable if sober.

Arthur E. Hertzler, 1870-1946

8   The greatest lesson in life is to know that even fools are right sometimes.

Winston C. Churchill, 1874-1965

9   What we do is a serious business; however, we must never take ourselves too seriously.

C. James Carrico, 1936-2002

10   She had spent all her life cutting, cutting, all her life had been blood and flesh. It is one of the tiresome but unavoidable facts about humanity that people cannot refresh themselves in the middle of their lives by a sudden, abrupt change of occupation.

Alexander Solzhenitsyn

11 Surgeons in general don't like theoretical or psychological problems. Things are either black or white. If they don't understand something, they try to put it out of their mind.

Charles Bosk

12 A true surgeon is like a South Dakota farmer who loses money year after year but when asked why he keeps farming, states "because that's what I am."

Gail Wadby

13 A trained surgeon knows how to do it; an educated surgeon knows why you do it.

Rodney Peyton

14 Curmudgeon is the guy who gets up at M+M, after you describe your brilliant save with an ER thoracotomy for GSW to the heart, and asks why you did not give prophylactic antibiotics.

Albert I. Alexander

15 Always pay attention to short surgeons!!!

Leo A. Gordon

16 The reversed curmudgeon is the guy who, after a case of total f***up is presented, stands up and asks whether an informed consent was taken or whether the patient was or was not hemophilic... or even better - whether the patient had a Swan Ganz inserted.

M. S.

17   Surgeons make the worst patients. Of course the opposite may also be true.

Karim Brohi

18   I wasn't God by a long shot, but as far as power was concerned, I was closer to Him than anyone else at hand.

William A. Nolen

19   Curmudgeon is also the guy who sees a video of a phenomenal new procedure in a conference and the moment the speaker completes his bit - expecting thunderous applause for his great act - he collars the mike and says, LOUDLY: "This... is grossly unethical! WHY did you show the patient's name in the slide?"

B. Ramana

20   In ancient Greece they believed in hubris and nemesis. These concepts seem to resonate with surgery. If you are arrogant or boastful [hubris] about your surgery, the next case that you operate upon will go horribly wrong [nemesis].

David Dent

21   My built in dogma detector: If someone prefaces their statement with "Always, always..." or "Never, never...", what they are then about to say is probably unsubstantiated dogma. If they use one of these two prefaces, and in addition poke the air with an index finger, assuming a stern face and focused glare - then it is pathognomonic of dogma.

David Dent

22 The great surgical lie: you go ahead; I'll meet you in the clinic later.

23 What is every surgeon's dream? To operate as well as he thinks he does. To earn as much money as everyone else thinks he does. To have as many affairs as his wife thinks he does.

24 A surgeon reaches maturity only when he stops taking himself too seriously. Some never reach this phase.

25 A surgeon is sometimes right, sometimes wrong, but never uncertain.

26 Pray to God but be sure to choose a good surgeon.

27 Drowning is a leading cause of death in surgeons: they think that they can walk on water, and when they sink, they can't keep their mouth shut.

73

Surgery & Love

1

The semen would appear, both from the smell and taste, to be a mawkish kind of substance, but when held some time in the mouth, it produces a warmth similar to spices, which lasts some time.

John Hunter, 1728-1793

2

[On romantic relationships between surgeons and nurses]: A good sheepdog does not kill in his own flock.

George Washington Crile, 1864-1943

74

Thyroid

1   It seems hardly credible that the loss of bodies so tiny as the parathyroids should be followed by a result so disastrous.

William Stewart Halsted, 1852-1922

2   As the result of needle biopsy to establish the diagnosis and the use of suppressive doses of thyroid hormone to treat benign goiters and struma lymphomatosa, and the use of corticosteroids to treat subacute thyroiditis, we have practically abolished thyroid surgery... the number of thyroid operations perfomed at the Cleveland Clinic fell from 2,700 in the year 1927 to less than 50 a year.

George Crile, Jr, 1907-1992

3   Recurrent laryngeal nerve damage produces voice changes, but not choking; they graduate in the choir from singing *Ave Maria* to *Old Man River*.

David Dent

4   Looking for the recurrent laryngeal nerve after previous thyroidectomy has all the sensitivity of detecting a landmine in Angola.

David Dent

5   His pre-op thyroid surgery counseling included: "Madam, this operation will make you hoarse and cough like a cow."

Dr. Frascani

75

Trauma, Emergency Room & War

1   When the guts are wounded, the whole body is griped and pined, the excrements come out at the wound, whereat often times the guts break forth with great violence.

Ambroise Paré,1510-1590

2   [About the inventor of gunpowder]: I think that the deviser of this deadly Engeine hath this for his recompense, that his name should be hidden by the darkness of perpetual ignorance, as not meriting for this, his most pernicious invention, any mention from posteriority.

Ambroise Paré,1510-1590

3   My practice in gunshot wounds has been a great measure different from all others, so that I have had the eyes of all the surgeons upon me, both on account of my suppos'd knowledge and method of treatment.

John Hunter, 1728-1793

4   Doctors will have more lives to answer for in the next world than even we generals.

Napoleon Bonaparte, 1769-1821

5   Wounds of the liver are very serious and despite most energetic treatment, the outcome is often regrettable.

Guillaume Dupuytren, 1777-1835

6   [Shock]... momentary pause in the act of death.

John Collins Warren, 1778-1856

7   [Shock]: The manifestation of the rude unhinging of the machinery of life.

Samuel Gross, 1805-1884

8   When he came to himself the splintered portions of his thigh bone had been extracted, the torn flesh cut away and the wound bandaged. Water was being sprinkled on his face. As soon as Prince Andrei opened his eyes the doctor bent down, kissed him on the lips with not a word and hurried away.

Leo Tolstoy, 1828-1910

9   War surgery can be very grim in the hands of untrained surgeons.

Ira A. Ferguson, 1896-1970

10   Though shock may be temporarily alleviated by transfusion, it cannot be arrested or overcome; resuscitation divorced from surgery is folly.

William Heneage Ogilvie, 1887-1971

11   That's why you call these forms of transportation donorcycles in Kentucky, where helmets are optional. Natural selection at work, although since you can get married here at age 13, most people have reproduced before they are pulled out of the gene pool.

Karen Draper

12   If you arrive in the ER and don't know what to do, start putting in tubes until somebody arrives who knows.

Rip Pfeiffer

13   A severe pelvic fracture is to be respected - there is little a surgeon can do to stop the bleeding, but much that can be done to make the bleeding worse.

Avery B. Nathens

14   Definition of a heavy trauma: somebody who arrives at the hospital in more than one ambulance.

John Edwards

15   In a case of hanging: cut the rope holding the victim and immediately loosen it from around the neck, unless the body is perfectly stiff-rigor mortis.

American Red Cross First Aid Text-Book, 1933

16   In urban trauma 'scoop and run' is better than 'stay and play'.

76

Truth

1   Truth is right and science is but a synonym to truth. Efficiency must acknowledge truth. Secrecy is the peculiar disease of efficiency. Publicity is the cure of the disease secrecy.

Ernest Amory Codman, 1869-1940

2   You have to report your complications truthfully to the point it hurts you.

Charles Drake, 1920-1998

3   In science, one never possesses the complete truth. One can only look for what, at a given time, cannot be proved wrong.

Daniel E. Lieberman

4   Truth, like surgery, may hurt, but it cures.

Han Suyin

5   The truth changes only slowly, and often in dubious company.

77

Unnecessary

1   Why dig a shaft 20 feet square through 60 or 70 feet of solid rock in order to bury a king? Yet today we still do the same thing. We spend $10,000 on a heart transplant and usually, from the stand point of the Welfare of Society, it is just about as productive as the shaft tombs were.

George Crile, Jr, 1907-1992

2   In America... when a patient asks you to take care of her, you will do everything within your power to cure her disease. Failing that, you will do everything within your power to prolong her life. And failing that, you will do everything within your power to relieve her suffering. The problem with that ethic is the word 'everything'. Everything may be unnecessary.

Alan Robert Spievack

3   The doctor is a person who still has his adenoid, tonsils, and appendix.

Lawrence J. Peter

4   The chief role for the measurement of gallbladder ejection fraction with a radioisoptope scan is to justify the performance of unnecessary laparoscopic cholecystectomies on perfectly normal gallbladders.

M. S.

5   Severe complications and deaths after ERCP are heartbreaking. But what is tragic is that in many such cases - in retrospect - it is clear that the original procedure was not really necessary.

M. S.

6   Never scope tomorrow what you can scope today.

78

Vessels

1   Embolectomy is doomed to failure unless you can demonstrate back-bleeding.

Ivor Lewis, 1895-1982

2   The entire gastrointestinal system to vascular surgeons is an incidental finding on the way to the aorta!

Leo A. Gordon

3   McDonald's 'breakfast for under a dollar' actually costs much more than that. You have to factor in the cost of coronary bypass surgery.

George Carlin

4   Pulling at the pulmonary artery causes tears... and TEARS.

Rick Paul

5   Why vascular surgeons do not like bowel surgery? Because shit does not clot.

6   One aspirin a day keeps the vascular surgeon away.

79

Wounds

1   If thou examinest a man having a gaping wound piercing through to his gullet; if he drinks water he chokes (and) it come out of the mouth of his wound; it is greatly inflamed, so that he develops fever from it; thou shouldst draw together that wound with stitching. Thou shouldst bind it with fresh meat the first day. Thou shouldst treat it afterward with grease, honey (and) lint every day, until he recovers. If , however, thou findst him continuing to have fever from that wound thou shouldst apply for him dry lint in the mouth of his wound, (and) moor (him) at his mooring stakes until he recovers.

Edwin Smith Papyru, written in Egypt, ~3000 years ago

2   One should not put fingers into a wound, but when other methods fail do not hesitate to apply pressure directly on the bleeding point. It is much better to have a live patient with a dirty wound than a dead patient with a clean wound.

American Red Cross First Aid Text-Book, 1933

3   I describe to my students what an injured animal does: it lies under a shady bush (rest, splint) by a water source (fluids, nutrition), licks the wound frequently (dressing changes) until it is clean and healing (time and patience) - and hope it makes them think past the gorgeous dressing promoted by manufacturers' reps.

Barry Alexander

4   When you deal with complicated wounds you get wound complications.

80

Writing & Publishing

1   [The advantages of precise bibliographic citations]: Several of the well known physicians and surgeons to whom I have given my book for proof reading and to edit especially for its prolixity have criticized me for my insistence on stating precisely the sources of my citations of other authors, by giving 'chapter and verse'. The answer gives my two reasons: 1. To make it easier for scholars to track down the sources. 2. As a result their comprehension of my text is better and clearer.

Henri de Mondeville, 1260-1320

2   No iron can stab the heart with such force as a period put just at the right place.

Isaac Babel, 1894-1941

3   For some strange reason the general opinion among doctors is that if one writes a book he must have superior knowledge of the subject. Since no one troubles to read the book the delusion is not discovered.

Arthur E. Hertzler, 1870-1946

4   The only one benefited by the writing of books is the one who writes them... but the financial compensation in medical writing is a negligible quantity.

Arthur E. Hertzler, 1870-1946

5   I think my cue in writing is to stick to the facts until I reach the point where my speculations will be of interest to the reader.

George Crile, Jr, 1907-1992

6　　The *New England Journal of Medicine* takes obvious observations and gives them statistical significance.

Richard Simmons

7　　[On writing]: I don't dawdle. I'm a surgeon. I make an incision, do what needs to be done and sew up the wound. There is a beginning, a middle and an end.

Richard Selzer

Index

Authors

Index

Subject

A

abdomen
> acute intestinal obstruction 4.1-4.3
> distension 4.4
> traumatic injuries 193.1
> washing-out 99.2
> when to operate 4.5, 110.11
> see also gastrointestinal tract

academics 2.1, 2.2

adenoids 199.3

administration/administrators 130.9, 153.4, 153.5, 154.7

alcohol
> effect on surgeons' performance 184.7
> pancreatitis and 145.4, 145.6
> as a stimulant 54.1

allergies 54.2

America
> surgery in 102.1, 102.2, 102.5
> unhealthiness of the diet 68.1, 201.3

amputation 6.1

anal cancer 34.1

anal fissures 34.2

anastomosis
> esophageal 180.11
> intestinal 68.3, 68.4, 105.4, 105.5

anatomy
> breast 29.1
> chest 8.2, 8.3, 8.6
> dissection 8.1, 172.2
> female 8.5
> and physiology 8.4

anesthesia
> bad signs 10.3, 10.4
> chloroform vs ether 10.1
> epidurals 10.6

anesthetists 10.2, 10.5, 139.5

animals
> practicing on 56.5, 163.2
> wounded 203.3

antibiotics
> efficacy of 94.5, 95.8, 95.10
> over-prescribing 96.13
> prophylaxis 95.7, 96.11
> resistance 96.12

appendicitis
> chronic 13.10
> diagnosis 13.8, 13.9, 14.12
> financial benefits to the surgeon 14.15
> function of the appendix 12.1
> medical treatment 13.7
> perforated 14.13
> surgeons' eagerness to operate 12.3, 14.11, 14.14, 199.3
> timing of appendectomy 12.2, 12.4-13.6, 14.13

art of medicine 16.1-16.4, 73.8

aspirin 201.6

assessment
> advantages 18.1, 50.2
> in an emergency 18.5
> fitness for the operation 18.7
> in hindsight 18.4
> radiology 18.3, 18.6, 19.8
> unnecessary 199.4-199.6
> when to avoid 18.2, 18.3

O

obesity 123.1, 150.6
    surgery for 123.2, 123.3
obstetricians 139.5
occupational change 184.10
old patients 127.1, 129.5
old surgeons
    breadth of knowledge 129.4
    cynicism of 129.2
    looking to retirement 129.1
    past their best 129.6-130.10
    and young surgeons 130.11
open-mindedness 112.1
operating technique
    daring 136.11
    dexterity 135.3, 135.5, 135.6
    ease of performance 135.7
    ignorance and 137.19, 137.20
    instruments 135.1, 136.8, 137.16
    keep it simple 137.17
    keyhole surgery 136.13
    Murphy's Law 137.15
    practicing 136.10
    six Ps 137.18
    suturing 136.12
    see also speed
operating theaters 132.3, 132.6, 133.10
    assistants 132.1, 132.5
    consumables 132.2, 133.9
    design 132.4
    schedules 133.8
    scrubbing up 133.11
    visitors 132.7

operations
    advisability 4.5, 74.13, 110.11
    inadvisability 42.1-42.3, 74.15, 81.1, 109.3
    Loeb's laws 139.3
orthopedics 140.8

P

pain
    operative 143.2
    prescribing analgesia 143.4
    suffered by doctors 143.1
    unavoidability 143.3
pancreas
    biopsy 146.7
    cancer 146.8, 146.9
    difficulty in operating on 145.2, 145.5
    pancreatitis 145.1, 145.3, 145.4, 145.6
parathyroid gland 191.1
parochialism 153.3
parotidectomy 136.9
pathology 148.1-148.4
patients
    care of 23.12, 157.5, 168.2
    and doctors 60.1, 150.1, 150.2, 150.4, 150.5,
    150.7
pelvic fractures 195.13
peptic ulcers 179.3-180.6
performance, surgery as 73.8
pericardiocentesis 83.5
peritonitis 97.17
pharmacists 54.5
physiology 8.4, 148.1, 148.2

Y